Let Us Demystify Lyme Disease

Finally, A Cookbook to Help You Eat Healthy and Help Reducing Unwanted Side Effects

BY

Stephanie Sharp

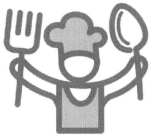

Copyright © 2019 by Stephanie Sharp

License Notes

Copyright 2019 by Stephanie Sharp All rights reserved.

No part of this Book may be transmitted or reproduced into any format for any means without the proper permission of the Author. This includes electronic or mechanical methods, photocopying or printing.

The Reader assumes all risk when following any of the guidelines or ideas written as they are purely suggestion and for informational purposes. The Author has taken every precaution to ensure accuracy of the work but bears no responsibility if damages occur due to a misinterpretation of suggestions.

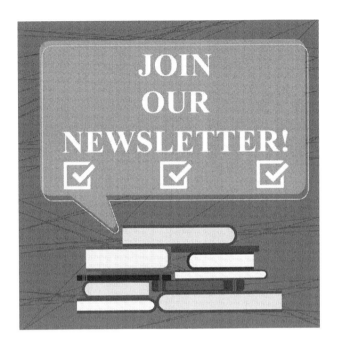

My deepest thanks for buying my book! Now that you have made this investment in time and money, you are now eligible for free e-books on a weekly basis! Once you subscribe by filling in the box below with your email address, you will start to receive free and discounted book offers for unique and informative books. There is nothing more to do! A reminder email will be sent to you a few days before the promotion expires so you will never have to worry about missing out on this amazing deal. Enter your email address below to get started. Thanks again for your purchase!

Table of Contents

Introduction 7

Loaded Sweet Potatoe Appetizers 10

Homemade Hummus 13

Spicy Herbal Tea 16

Kimchi 18

Sunflower Seed Salad 21

Baked Salmon Topped with Fresh Mango Salsa 24

Stuffed Eggplants 27

Coconut, Fruit and Granola Breakfast 30

Poppy Seed, Lemon and Coconut Muffins 32

Lettuce Wraps 35

Warm Milk with Cinnamon 38

Apricots Health Bars 40

Cilantro and Citrus Chicken Spread 42

Mushrooms and Herbs Risotto 44

Taco Style Dip.. 47

Tuna and Avocado Salad... 50

Crispy Zucchini Chips... 53

Quinoa tortillas... 55

Berry and Almond Sorbet 57

Ground Beef 59

Chicken with Herbs... 61

Chicken Soup with Greens.. 64

Enchilada Casserole 67

Healthy and Delicious Chicken Fingers 70

Gluten and Sugar Free Bread Buns 73

Conclusion 76

About the Author 78

Author's Afterthoughts 79

Introduction

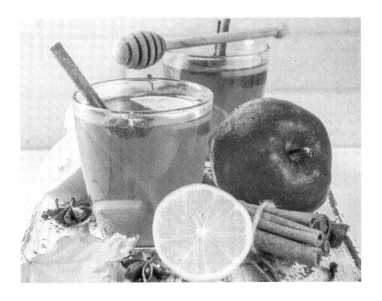

Let us explain briefly, what the Lyme disease is all about. Firstly, you must know that the disease will more than likely develop after you have been bitten by a tick. That is why it is so important that if you do notice and feel a bite that you observe the area and quickly seek medical attention.

You will normally notice a rash around the bite, like a small bull's eye. Experiencing itchiness or even pain in the affected area.

Unfortunately, some untreated tick bites can degenerate and cause severe illness. You could also experience headaches, fever, vomiting, as the Lyme disease will eventually attack the membrane around your brain if no medical care is sought. In some cases, it can cause joint pain as well as the destruction of some of the digestive lining. This is a serious matter and anyone who is bitten by a tick should always consult medical professionals.

Okay, now that you know that Lyme disease is much more serious than initially believed, if you are a Lyme disease victim, your life is not over. Don't worry, you are not alone. However, t you should get as educated as possible on the subject, including the new diet you will have to adopt, at least temporarily until the Lyme disease can be treated or controlled.

Overall, you will want to cut gluten from your diet, eliminate most dairy products and sugars. This will help reduce any type of inflammation might be experiencing though out your body. You will cook simple meals with simple basic ingredients to be able to prevent your body working too hard to digest your meals. You will then protect your digestive system and keep all the needed energy to keep going throughout the day. You will detoxify your body on a regular basis, keeping your organs as healthy as possible and eliminating any harsh chemicals. No processed foods should be included in this diet.

We will explain in detail in the conclusion what foods you should include in your new lifestyle, to help you feel good for as possible.

Loaded Sweet Potatoe Appetizers

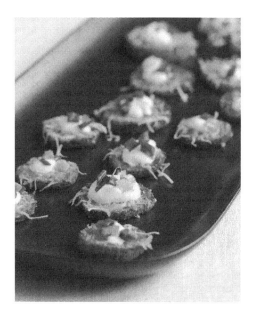

We see the use of sweet potatoes increasing on the menus of restaurants and there is a good reason for it. They are more nutritional than regular white potatoes, and in my opinion tastier! They are an excellent source of vitamin A, that will help your immune system.

Servings: 4

Preparation time: 50 minutes

Ingredients:

- 4 sweet potatoes
- ½ cup roasted pine nuts
- 3 cups fresh chopped kale
- ½ tsp. garlic powder
- ½ tsp. onion powder
- 2 Tbsp. unsalted butter (room temperature)
- Salt, black pepper
- 2/3 cup crumbled Goat cheese

Method:

1. Preheat the oven to 400 degrees F.
2. In the microwave cook the potatoes one at a time for 3-4 minutes each.
3. You should cook them enough to be able to cut them and remove some of the flesh form the middle.
4. In a mixing bowl, combine the butter with the kale, spices and goat cheese. Add the cooked sweet potatoes you remove and mix again.
5. Fill each sweet potato with the mixture and sprinkle with pine nuts.
6. On a grease baking sheet, place the potatoes and bake in the oven for 30-40 minutes.
7. Serve warm.

Homemade Hummus

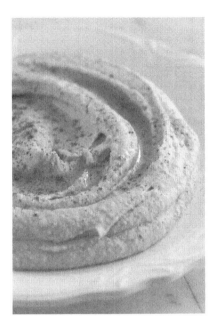

Hummus is a very popular food item these days. People will use it as a dip or even as condiment in their sandwiches. Manufacturers have started making them with added ingredients, such as roasted peppers, black beans, olives or even edamame. We are going back to the simple recipe, but you will benefit from the nutritional value of the chickpea. They are loaded with vitamin B6 and this will also give a boost to your defense system.

Servings: 3-4

Preparation time: 20 minutes

Ingredients:

- ¼ cup olive oil
- 3 Tbsp. lemon juice
- 2 cans chickpeas, well rinsed and drained
- 1 tbsp. minced garlic
- ¼ tsp. smoked paprika
- ¼ tsp. dried cumin
- Salt, black pepper

Method:

1. You can use a high-speed blender or a food processor for this recipe, it's up to you. I think both do a great job.
2. First, add half of the oil, chickpeas and lemon juice. Activate the blending machine until it is reduced into puree.
3. Add the garlic and spices and activate again until the mixture is very smooth.
4. Serve with ray veggies, such as celery, broccoli, cauliflower.
5. You can keep this hummus in the refrigerator up to a week.

Spicy Herbal Tea

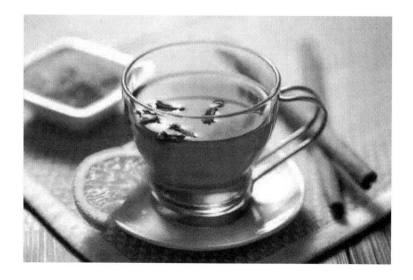

Lately, it has been brought to people's attention that spices can also impact your health in a positive way. Turmeric is one of them. This spice has some anti-inflammatory properties that can help you if you are diagnosed with the Lyme diseases. Using it in your tea is one good idea, also I often use it in my smoothies.

Servings: 2

Preparation time: 20 minutes

Ingredients:

- 2 Tbsp. agave syrup
- 1 tsp. dried turmeric
- ½ tsp. ground nutmeg
- ½ tsp. ground ginger
- 2 cups water
- 2 tea bags (your favorite, I prefer green or black tea for this recipe)
- 1 cup almond milk

Method:

1. Bring the water to boil in a medium saucepan and infuse the tea bags for 7-8 minutes.
2. Remove the bags and keep on low temperature.
3. Add the spices, agave syrup and the almond milk.
4. Stir in all ingredients mix well and let it simmer for another 10 minutes
5. Serve into 2 tea cups.

Kimchi

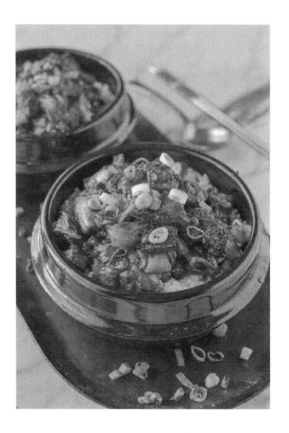

The fermentation process of Kimchi produces a good type of bacteria in your stomach. This will help your digestion and your overall health. We will explain how to proceed below.

Servings: 3-4

Preparation time: a few hours +

Ingredients:

- 1 head of green cabbage
- 1 large peeled and shredded carrot
- 2 minced green onions
- 1 tbsp. minced garlic
- 1 tbsp. brown sugar
- 2 Tbsp. sesame oil
- 1 Tbsp. sesame seeds
- 1 tbsp. Worcestershire sauce
- 1 tbsp. rice vinegar
- 1 minced jalapeno pepper
- 1 tbsp. chili powder

Method:

1. Preheat the oven to 400 degrees F.
2. If you can plan to make this recipe ahead and let is ferment overnight, that is great, if not, plan to let it ferment for at least few hours.
3. Use a grater or other culinary tool you like to shred the cabbage and carrot. I like to make it as fine as possible. When cutting the jalapeno, I highly suggest wearing gloves, so you don't get some on your skin.
4. Place the veggies (garlic, onions, carrot, jalapeno and cabbage) sin a large air tight container.
5. In a mixing bowl, combine the oil, sauce, vinegar, spices and brown sugar and add to the veggies. Stir very well.
6. Place in the refrigerator.
7. Meanwhile, place the sesame seeds on a baking sheet and toast them. Watch them closely so they do not burn.
8. Add to the cabbage mixture and put back in the refrigerator.
9. Once it has been a few hours or more, taste the cabbage and serve as side dish or even in your sandwiches as topping.

Sunflower Seed Salad

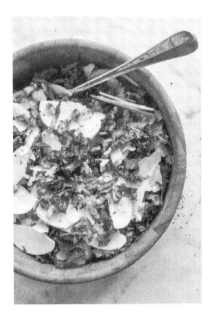

You can now buy sunflower seed everywhere, even without the shells and use them in many dishes, including your salads. This fresh and colorful salad is a perfect lunch any day.

Servings: 3-4

Preparation time: 20 minutes

Ingredients:

- 1 large sliced avocado
- 1 large sliced red bell pepper
- ¼ cup diced red onion
- 4 cups spinach baby leaves
- 1 Tbsp. lime juice
- 3 tbsp. roasted unsalted sunflower seeds
- 1 Tbsp. balsamic vinegar
- 2 Tbsp. olive oil
- ½ Tbsp. Dijon mustard
- ½ tsp. garlic powder
- Salt, black pepper

Method:

1. In a mixing bowl, combine the oil, vinegar, mustard, lime juice, garlic powder, salt, pepper.
2. Slice the pepper and after removing the pit form the avocado, also slice it. You can choose to dice to slice the red onion, it's your choice.
3. Divide the spinach leave into 4 plates and add some red pepper, avocado and sprinkle some diced onion and sunflower seeds.
4. Then, add some vinaigrette on each plate to your taste.

Baked Salmon Topped with Fresh Mango Salsa

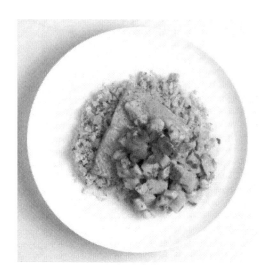

Salmon is so good for you for many reasons It contains some omega-3 fatty acids and it can help you also reduce the inflammation your experiencing in your body. Enjoy it with a sweet and tangy mango salsa.

Servings: 4

Preparation time: 50 minutes

Ingredients:

- 4 medium size salmon fillets
- 1 fresh mango
- 1 cup diced fresh tomatoes
- 1 tbsp. minced cilantro
- 1 tbsp. minced fresh parsley
- 1 tbsp. lemon juice
- 1 tbsp. olive oil
- Salt, black pepper
- 1 tbsp. Chili powder

Method:

1. Preheat the oven to 350 degrees F.
2. Grease with olive oil a baking dish and set aside for now.
3. Get all the ingredients out. On your kitchen counter.
4. Peel and dice the mango, the tomatoes and minced the fresh herbs.
5. In a mixing bowl. Combine the oil, spices, lemon juice.
6. Add the fruits and herbs and mix well.
7. Season the salmon with salt and pepper on both sides and place on baking dish.
8. Add the mango topping on each salon filet and bake for 30 minutes or so.

Stuffed Eggplants

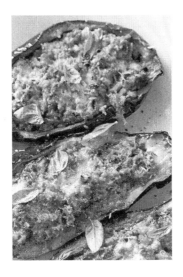

In this recipe, we will play with 2 ingredients that are very good for your diet if you are dealing with Lyme disease. Beans and eggplant are the core ingredients in this recipe. You will love how the beans' topping we created will enhance the flavor of the eggplant. Enjoy!

Servings: 4

Preparation time: 60 minutes

Ingredients:

- 1 large eggplant
- Salt, black pepper
- ½ tsp. dried cumin
- 1 tbsp. olive oil
- 1 cup shredded mozzarella cheese
- 1 cup cooked black beans
- 1 tbsp. minced garlic
- 4 sliced bacon

Method:

1. Preheat the oven to 400 degrees F.
2. Grease a large baking sheet.
3. Cut the eggplant in half and place face down on the baking sheet.
4. Put in the oven for 30 minutes.
5. Meanwhile, cook the bacon in a frying pan. Remove the bacon once cooked but keep the bacon grease.
6. You can fry the garlic in it for 5 minutes.
7. Then, combine the crumbled bacon, cheese, garlic, beans and seasonings in a mixing bowl.
8. Remove the eggplant form the oven and turn it over.
9. Top it off with the mixture you just created.
10. Place aback in the oven for another 15 minutes or until the cheese has melted completely.

Coconut, Fruit and Granola Breakfast

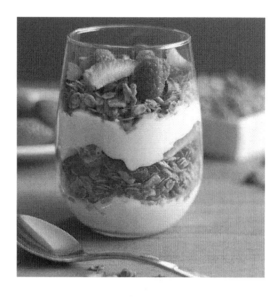

Don't pour yourself a large bowl of sugary cereals first thing in the morning, this will not help your health condition at all. No need to eat eggs and every day either. Choose a lighter breakfast version like this one and enjoy the freshness of the chosen ingredients.

Servings: 2-3

Preparation time: 15 minutes

Ingredients:

- 1/3 cup fresh blueberries
- 1 large sliced banana
- ¼ cup sliced almonds
- 2 cups cottage cheese
- 2 tbsp. flaxseeds
- ¼ cup roasted shredded coconut

Method:

1. Get your serving bowls out.
2. Divide the cottage cheese equally.
3. Add some fruits, flaxseeds, almonds and shredded coconut to each bowl.
4. Serve!

Poppy Seed, Lemon and Coconut Muffins

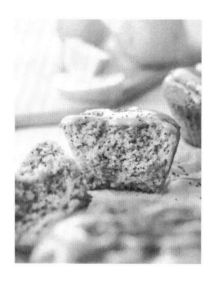

Poppy seeds and lemon go together like peas and carrots. However, once you will have tasted the addition of coconut flavor in this recipe, you will think of these 3 ingredients as inseparable from now on. I recommend using a mixture of almond and coconut flour, but if you prefer, you can use only almond and add coconut flakes instead.

Servings: 6-8

Preparation time: 50 minutes

Ingredients:

- 2 cups coconut flour
- Pinch salt
- ½ tsp. cinnamon
- 1 tbsp. poppy seeds
- ½ tsp. baking soda
- 1 tbsp. lemon juice
- 1 tbsp. lemon zest
- 2 tbsp. coconut, milk
- ½ tsp. baking powder
- ½ tsp. vanilla extract
- 1 tbsp. coconut oil (room temperature)
- 1 large egg

Method:

1. Preheat the oven to 350 degrees F.
2. Grease a muffin tin and set aside for now.
3. In a large mixing bowl, combine the dry Ingredients: coconut flour, salt, cinnamon, baking soda, baking powder, poppy seeds.
4. In a different bowl, combine the wet Ingredients: coconut oil, egg, vanilla, coconut milk, lemon juice and lemon zest.
5. Add the wet mixture to the dry one.
6. Pour the muffin mixture into the muffin holes and bake for 40 minutes.
7. Wait until they have cooled down a little before eating.

Lettuce Wraps

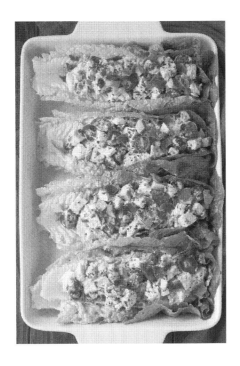

Again, this is also a popular trend. We want to eliminate breads and carbs form your diet as much as possible, so opting for lettuce leaves as wraps is genius. In this recipe, we will not add meat, however you are welcome to add grilled chicken, roasted turkey or even sautéed tofu if you want a little protein in your meal. But for now, let's enjoy this veggies' medley.

Servings: 4

Preparation time: 30 minutes

Ingredients:

- 8 large lettuce leaves (romaine lettuce works well for this or Iceberg if you prefer)
- ¼ diced yellow onion
- 1 Tbsp. minced garlic
- 2 medium sliced zucchinis
- ¼ cup sliced black olives
- Salt, black pepper
- 1 tbsp. unsalted butter
- Dressing
- 4 Tbsp. sour cream
- 1 cup ricotta cheese
- 1 Tbsp. chili powder
- 1 Tbsp. minced fresh cilantro
- Salt, Black pepper

Method:

1. In a frying pan, sautéed the garlic, onions and sliced zucchinis together in butter. Season with salt and pepper.
2. In a mixing bowl, prepare the dressing by missing the ricotta cheese, sour cream, chili powder and cilantro.
3. Use 2 large leaves per person and add a generous portion of the veggie's mixture and top it off with the dressing and sliced black olives.

Warm Milk with Cinnamon

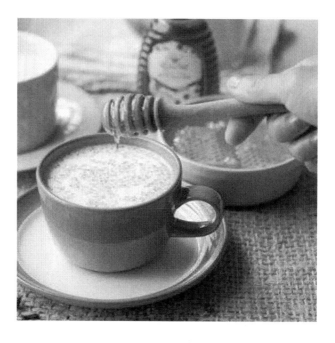

We talked about the addition of certain spices in your beverages, to give you a health boost. Turmeric was one of them. Cinnamon can also help your body facilitate the digestion, lowering your blood sugar levels, even reducing the risks of heart diseases and some cancers.

Servings: 2

Preparation time: 15 minutes

Ingredients:

- 2 cups coconut milk
- ½ cup half and half cream
- 1 Tbsp. maple syrup
- 1 tsp. cinnamon
- Pinch nutmeg

Method:

- In a medium saucepan, combine the crema and coconut milk.
- Add the spices and the maple syrup.
- Stir well to combine, keep on low temperature until ready to serve.
- You can add a little roasted coconut on top when serving if you like.

Apricots Health Bars

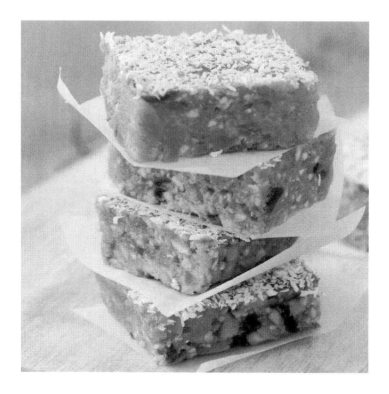

You don't find many recipes that contain apricot. However, because it is a beneficial food item, which we listed it in the last chapter, we recommend you try to add it in your cobblers or homemade low carbs desserts. This recipe will also let you add some seeds and/or nuts. Enjoy fully!

Servings: 8-10

Preparation time: 45 minutes

Ingredients:

- 2 cups unsweetened shredded coconut flakes
- 2 tbsp. flaxseeds
- ½ unsalted cup pumpkin seeds
- 1 cup gluten free rolled oats
- 2/3 cup chopped dried apricots
- ½ cup agave syrup
- 4 tbsp. coconut oil (room temperature)
- Pinch salt

Method:

1. Preheat the oven to 350 degrees F.
2. Grease a square baking dish and set aside.
3. In a saucepan, combine the diced apricots and 2 tablespoons of coconut oil with agave syrup. Cook for about 15 minutes on medium heat.
4. In a mixing bowl, combine the rest of the coconut oil with the oats and the salt, flax seeds and pumpkin seeds.
5. Press firmly this mixture on the bottom of the dish.
6. Add the apricot's mixture on top.
7. Bake the dessert for about 3 5minutes and let it cool down before cutting into squares.

Cilantro and Citrus Chicken Spread

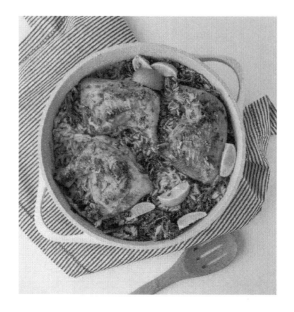

Lime and lemon are welcome in your diet. You can make some yummy lemonade, or you can also incorporate the fruits into many other dishes. Let's make some lime and cilantro chicken salad you can spread on your fresh avocados or rice crackers.

Servings: 2-3

Preparation time: 15 minutes

Ingredients:

- 2 cans of cooked shredded chicken.
- 3 Tbsp... cup mayonnaise
- 1 Tbsp. Minced fresh cilantro
- 1 tbsp. lemon juice
- 1 minced green onion
- Salt, black pepper
- Smoke paprika
- Avocado or ice crackers to serve it on

Method:

1. This recipe is very easy to make.
2. Make sure you drain carefully the chicken form any juice.
3. Place in a mixing bowl and add the mayonnaise, spices and all other ingredients.
4. Use a fork to mix well.
5. We suggest using it on avocados or rice crackers, but you can also fill a lettuce leave and have chicken salad lettuce wrap.

Mushrooms and Herbs Risotto

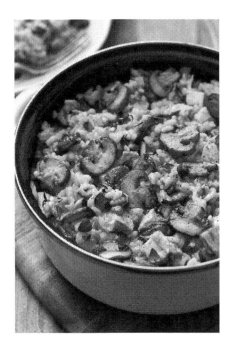

My son loves mushrooms and I always try to find recipes that accommodate them nicely. Risotto is a wonderful grain, and conscious of the Lyme disease, it can be a great option. I love to choose the freshest herbs, and I try to change it up from time to time.

Servings: 3-4

Preparation time: 45 minutes

Ingredients:

- 3 cups fresh button sliced mushrooms
- 1 tbsp. minced fresh parsley
- 1 tbsp. fresh minced basil
- 1 tbsp. minced fresh oregano
- 1 chopped leek
- 2 minced cloves garlic
- 2 tbsp. olive oil
- 3 cups Vegetables broth
- 1 ½ cup Risotto uncooked grains
- Salt, black pepper

Method:

1. Boil the vegetables broth and once it is boiling add the uncooked risotto grains.
2. Keep cooking on medium heat for about 15 minutes and then turn on the stove burner, cover the saucepan and let it rest some more.
3. Meanwhile, you need to chop the leek, garlic, all fresh herbs and mushrooms.
4. Heat olive oil in a frying pan and sautéed the veggies together for about 10-12 minutes.
5. Once the risotto is cooked, add the cooked veggies, combine and season with salt and pepper.
6. Taste before serving and adjust the seasonings if needed.

Taco Style Dip

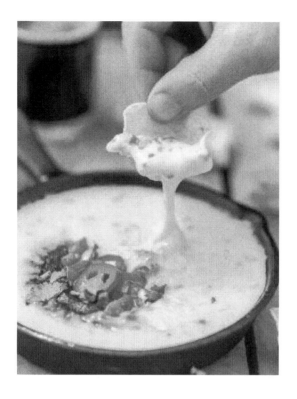

Beans are an excellent source of proteins and can be added to many dishes. Think about adding them to your meatloaf's, salads, or stews. This time, we will make a special dip including beans and veggies in layers, making it yummy and beautiful at the same time. This dip is as beautiful as it is tasty, I promise!

Servings: 4

Preparation time: 30 minutes

Ingredients:

- 2 can red kidney beans, well rinsed and drained
- 1 cup diced fresh tomatoes
- 1 large pitted avocado
- 1 tsp. lemon juice
- Salt, black pepper
- 1 minced green onion
- ¾ cup sour cream
- ½ tsp. chili powder

Method:

1. You need to use some clear small plastic cups for this recipe to get the full effect.
2. In a mixing bowl, combine the beans and sour cream with the chili powder.
3. In a separate bowl, mash the avocado with lemon juice and salt and pepper.
4. Then, mince your onion and dice your fresh tomatoes.
5. Now, start layering your dip in each individual cup.
6. Line up the 4 cups and fill each of them to about 1/3 with the sour cream mixture.
7. Next, add a nice layer of the mashed avocado mixture.
8. Next, add some diced tomatoes and minced onion as topping.
9. Serve this fabulous dip with some rice cracker or natural corn chips.
10. You can add some additional topping such as sliced jalapenos or sliced black olives.
11. You can also add it on your plate when you are serving tacos or fajitas, people will just love it.

Tuna and Avocado Salad

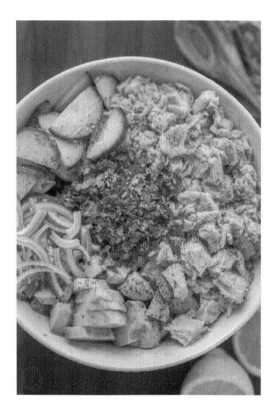

I love making this salad with fresh tuna but if all you have is canned, then you can still make a delicious and healthy salad. I also love to add crumbled bacon pieces in this salad to add some yummy saltiness to the dish. Then, try to add some eye catching colors such as red onion, red bell peppers or even sundried tomatoes.

Servings: 4

Preparation time: 20 minutes

Ingredients:

- 2 -3 cans white tuna, well drained
- 1 large pitted avocado diced
- 4 slices turkey bacon
- 1 can white kidney beans, well rinsed and drained
- ½ cup sliced radishes
- 1 cup fresh sliced mushrooms
- 4 cups arugula lettuce leaves

Dressing:

- 4 tbsp. avocado oil
- 1 minced green onion
- 1 Tbsp. white balsamic vinegar
- ½ tsp. garlic powder
- ½ tsp. cumin
- 1 tbsp. poppy seeds
- 1 tbsp. Dijon mustard

Method:

1. In a mixing bowl., combine all the ingredients listed for the dressing. Set aside.
2. Cook the turkey in the microwave for 5 minutes. Let it cool down and crumble.
3. Prepare the veggies and prepare the plating.
4. Divide the arugula in 4 plates. Add some diced avocado, mushrooms and radishes.
5. Also sprinkle crumbled turkey bacon.
6. Top it off with generous portion of white tuna.
7. Finish by pouring some dressing on each plate.

Crispy Zucchini Chips

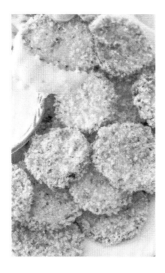

You do not want to include potato chips in your diet. But you might want to create some crispy snacks to eat with your sandwiches. Crispy zucchinis as we propose below, can perfectly replace a side with some of your entrees. They can also be a great afternoon snacks also when you are just a little hungry.

Servings: 3-4

Preparation time: 45 minutes

Ingredients:

- 2 medium zucchinis sliced
- 2 medium eggs
- ¼ cup shredded Parmesan cheese
- ½ cup coconut flour
- 1 Tbsp. coconut oil (room temperature)
- Salt, black pepper
- Pinch smoked paprika

Method:

1. Preheat the oven to 400 degrees F.
2. In a mixing bowl, combine the parmesan cheese with the coconut flour and spices.
3. In a different bowl, whisk the eggs.
4. Slice the zucchini very thin.
5. Grease a baking sheet with coconut oil.
6. Take each zucchini slice and dip it in the whisked eggs, then in the coconut flour mixture.
7. Place all the zucchini slices on the baking dish.
8. Cook in the oven for 30 minutes, until you are satisfied how crispy they are. You can repeat if you have more zucchini slices.

Quinoa tortillas

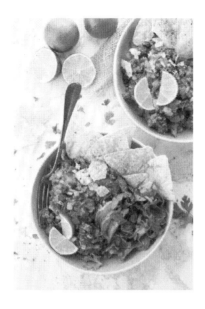

You will be eliminating most of your intake of high carb foods, like bread and pasta. But because we all love fajitas, tacos and sandwiches, it is interesting to be able to create a substitute for the regular tortilla. Using quinoa is a fabulous idea because quinoa is so rich in natural proteins, fibers and antioxidants.

Servings: 2-3

Preparation time: 30 minutes

Ingredients:

- 3 cups quinoa flour
- ½ cup brown rice flour
- Pinch salt
- 1 Tbsp. unsalted butter
- ¾ cup hot water

Method:

1. This is a simple recipe.
2. In a large mixing bowl, combine both flours and the water with salt.
3. Form a dough ball and use a rolling pin to roll some nice and even tortillas.
4. Heat the butter in pan and cook the tortillas until done. (a minute or so on each side)
5. Note that you can certainly add some flour or water as needed to get the desired texture for your dough.

Berry and Almond Sorbet

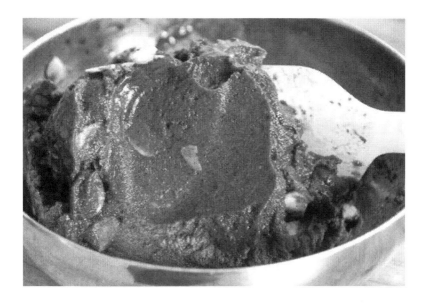

I used to always order sorbet as a young kid instead of ice cream from the ice cream shop. As I grow older, I totally understand why I preferred sorbet. It is so much more refreshing, delicious and a healthier. Let's make one with the fresh berries of your choice and almond milk.

Servings: 2-3

Preparation time: 1 hour

Ingredients:

- 1 cup almond milk
- ½ tsp. almond extract
- 1 medium banana
- ¼ cup blueberries
- ¼ cup strawberries
- ½ tsp. lemon juice

Method:

1. Proceed to freeze your fruits ahead: banana, blueberries and strawberries.
2. Then, add all of them after slicing the strawberries and bananas into the food processor.
3. Add the almond milk, lemon juice and almond extract.
4. Continue blending until the texture is very smooth and thick.
5. You can eat right away when you are satisfied with the texture or you can place back in individual cups in the freezer if you think it needs to be slightly more frozen.
6. You can also add some roasted coconut on top.

Ground Beef

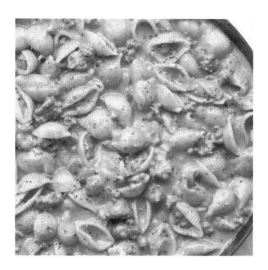

You will enjoy the improved taste of the grass-fed ground beef. However, it may be difficult for you to acquire locally, or maybe your budget will mean you cannot purchase it all the time, especially if you are cooking for a large family. If you are able to use this meat in a casserole or tacos, you can go with regular lean meat, like Turkey. However, you will taste the different in this dish.

Servings: 2-3

Preparation time: 30 minutes

Ingredients:

- 1-pound fresh grass fed ground beef
- 1 tbsp. minced garlic
- 1 tbsp. minced fresh parsley
- 1 tbsp. minced fresh basil
- 1 tsp. Worcestershire sauce
- Salt, black pepper
- Little olive oil

Method:

1. Remove your meat out of the refrigerator and let it sit out for 10 minutes so it's not too cold.
2. Heat some olive oil and cook the garlic first for a few minutes.
3. Add the meat and the fresh herbs as well as the Worcestershire sauce.
4. Season with salt and pepper.
5. Stir constantly to make sure the meta stays crumbly. Keep the temperature to a medium heat.
6. It should take about 15-minutes or so for the meat to be done.
7. You can serve as is or with a side of low fat sour cream.

Chicken with Herbs

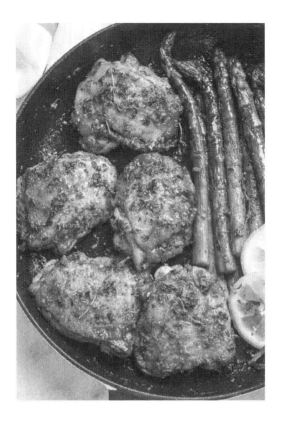

Chicken should not be underestimated. It is certainly a healthy choice if you are dealing with Lyme disease. Here, it is recommended you use free range chicken, as it is healthier and free from hormones. You will not regret it.

Servings: 4

Preparation time: 1 hour

Ingredients:

- 4 chicken breasts or chicken tights (choose hormone free if you can or as they call it free range) – leave the skin on
- Grapeseed oil
- 1 tbsp. Italian seasonings
- ½ cup chopped sundried tomatoes
- 1 cup sour cream
- Salt, black pepper
- 1 tsp. chili powder

Method:

1. Preheat the oven to 375 degrees F.
2. Grease a baking dish and set aside for now.
3. Place the chosen chicken skin facing up on the baking dish.
4. Brush grapeseed oil generously on all the chicken (skin).
5. Sprinkle the Italian seasonings all over the chicken and bake in the oven for an hour or so.
6. Meanwhile, prepare a side sauce for it.
7. In a mixing bowl, combine the sour cream with the chopped sundried tomatoes, salt, pepper and chili powder.
8. Serve on the side with the baked chicken.

Chicken Soup with Greens

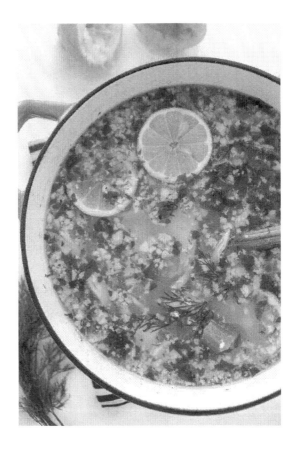

If you are creating a bouillon from scratch, you will benefit from the extra collagen the chicken bones will give you, so I recommended it. Then, also use some very valuable green vegetables to add to your soup and of course the right herbs and spices.

Servings: 4

Preparation time: 45 minutes

Ingredients:

- 6 cups low fat low salt chicken broth (even better if you baked a chicken and you can make your own broth)
- 3 cups shredded cooked chicken (left over baked chicken or rotisserie chicken works well)
- 2 cups fresh baby spinach leaves
- 2 chopped celery stalks
- 1 tbsp. minced fresh parsley
- 1 tbsp. fresh minced rosemary
- Salt, black pepper
- 1 tbsp. minced garlic
- 1 small chopped yellow onion
- 1 tbsp. unsalted butter

Method:

1. In a large saucepan, heat the butter on medium heat. Sautéed the garlic, onion and celery for 6-7 minutes. Add the herbs and then the chicken broth.
2. Bring to boil.
3. Add the baby spinach leaves and cook for 5 minutes.
4. Turn down the heat to low temperature and add the cooked chicken and rest of seasonings.
5. Let it simmer for at least 30 minutes or until ready to serve.

Enchilada Casserole

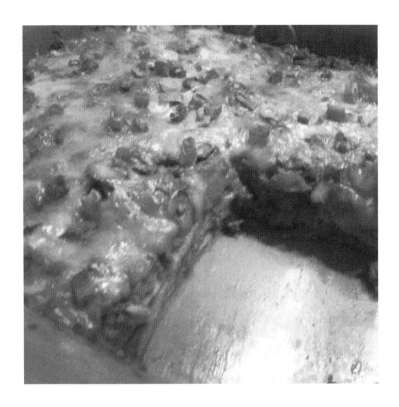

Is this a lasagna? Is this a Mexican casserole? What is it exactly you might ask? It is what you want to make of it. I personally call it the deluxe enchilada casserole. Get ready for an explosion of flavors with a wise choice of ingredients. We keep this dish gluten free and dairy free.

Servings: 4-6

Preparation time: 60 minutes

Ingredients:

- 1 package of the small corn tortillas (make sure they are as natural as possible, no added sugars or flavors).
- 1 large can refried beans (from health food store)
- 1 medium sliced yellow onion
- 1 diced jalapeno pepper
- 1 tbsp. olive oil
- 1 1/2 cup shredded Monterey Jack cheese
- Enchilada sauce
- ½ tsp. garlic powder
- ½ tsp. onion powder
- ½ tbsp. dried cumin
- ½ tsp. dried oregano
- Salt, black pepper
- 2 cups vegetables broth (low sodium0
- 2 tbsp. tomato pasta
- 1 tbsp. rice vinegar

Method:

1. Preheat the oven to 350 degrees F.
2. Grease a rectangle baking dish and set aside.
3. Let's prepare the enchilada sauce first.
4. In a medium saucepan, bring to boil the vegetates broth.
5. Add the tomato pasta, vinegar and all seasonings.
6. Stir constantly until the sauce becomes thicker.
7. If it does not, you can add a little rice flour to it to help.
8. Once you are satisfied with the texture and the teats (you should make sure the seasonings are perfect), you can reduce the temperature to low.
9. In a frying pan, heat the olive oil and cook the onion and jalapeno pepper for 5 minutes.
10. Now, it will be time to assemble your casserole.
11. Use a layer of corn bread tortillas on the bottom of the dish.
12. Add a generous layer of refried beans and top if off with some enchilada sauce. Add another layer of corn tortillas, refried bean and sauce.
13. Finally, add a layer of the shredded cheese.
14. Now you can bake this casserole for 45 minutes in the oven or even the cheese is melted and golden.

Healthy and Delicious Chicken Fingers

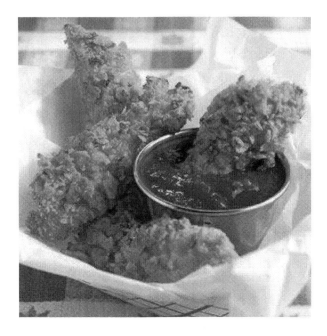

There is no way that you are never craving some chicken nuggets or chicken tenders. Everyone loves them. You simply must learn to make them with the proper and acceptable ingredients regarding the Lyme diseases condition. Here we go, follow our lead!

Servings: 3-4

Preparation time: 40 minutes

Ingredients:

- 1-pound chicken tenderloins (organic or not)
- ½ cup coconut flour
- 1 cup rice flour
- 2 large eggs
- 1 tbsp. coconut milk
- Salt, black pepper
- ½ tsp. garlic powder
- ½ tsp. onion powder
- ½ tsp. cayenne pepper
- Coconut oil for frying

Method:

1. Make sure you clean and cut the chicken tenderloins as needed, if the pieces are too big.
2. In a mixing bowl, combine the coconut flour, rice flour, onion powder garlic powder, cayenne pepper, salt and black pepper.
3. In a second bowl, whisk the eggs and the coconut milk together.
4. Heat the coconut oil in a large frying pan.
5. Use your hands (you can wear gloves if you like) and dip each chicken tenderloin one by one in the eggs mixture and then the flour mixture.
6. Place the chicken tenderloins in the hot coconut oil and fry for about 7-8 minutes on each side.
7. Remove and let the extra oil get absorbed on paper towels before serving.
8. If you want to make a quick dipping sauce, combine sour cream with minced garlic and minced chives, you will love it!

Gluten and Sugar Free Bread Buns

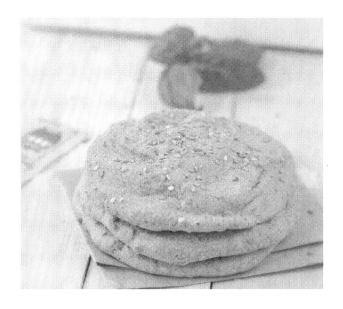

Let's prepare some buns that are free of almost everything potentially harmful to your health but taste fantastic and are convenient to use for meals. That's right, this recipe is dairy free, gluten free and sugar free. That's incredible, let's start working on them so you can start eating them more often as recommended.

Servings: 4-6

Preparation time: 60 minutes+

Ingredients:

- 1 cup brown rice flour
- 1 cup tapioca flour
- 1 Tbsp. agave syrup
- 2 tsp. xanthan gum
- 1 tbsp. instead yeast
- ¼ cup egg whites
- ½ tsp. salt
- 2/3 cup soy milk
- 2 Tbsp. olive oil

Method:

1. In a bowl, combine the rice flour and tapioca flour. Add the xanthan gum and the agave syrup as well as the yeast and salt.
2. Take a wooden spoon and mix well and set aside for now.
3. In a different bowl now using an electric mixer beat the egg's whites with the oil and the soy milk. Mix until the mixture is nice and fluffy.
4. Add all the dried ingredients form your previous mixture into the egg whites' mixture.
5. Using the electric mixer once more, activate for a few minutes.
6. You should be left with a nice lumps free dough, but a dough that still needs to rise.
7. Dump this dough into large muffin tin holes, after greasing the pan of course.
8. Let the dough rise for about 45 minutes.
9. Preheat the oven to 350 degrees F.
10. Bake the buns you just prepare for about 15-18 minutes.
11. They will make perfect buns for burgers, sandwiches, and more.

Conclusion

So, you might wonder what you can eat exactly when on a diet because suffering Lyme disease. Since you must eliminate gluten, you should have excluded pasta, white bread and white rice, but you can certainly include millet, quinoa, brown rice, corn or buckwheat.

When it's time to choose your veggies, you will have plenty of options, but stay away from the ones that are starchy. All green leafy vegetables are an excellent choice, such as lettuce, spinach, kale, arugula, green collards. You can also include green beans, carrots, squash, leeks, shallots, zucchini, broccoli, cauliflower, asparagus, artichoke, celery, onion, parsnips, cabbage, mushrooms, peppers, tomatoes, sweet potatoes, eggplants and cucumber.

Now, let's choose the appropriate fruits you may use, shall we? You can choose banana, orange, berries, lemon, lime, grapefruit, coconut, grapes, cherries, grapes, apples and avocado. As far as proteins and meats, here are the foods you should add to your grocery cart: eggs, black beans, lentils, kidney beans, pinto beans, fish (tilapia, sole, salmon), lamb, chicken, pork, crab, lobster, turkey, sausages, beef and buffalo.

Add also some seeds and nuts to your diet such as sunflower seeds, almonds, Brazil nuts, chia seeds, peanuts, hemp seeds, cashews, pumpkin seeds, sesame seeds, flax seeds, and walnuts.

We certainly hope you have enjoyed our cookbook and are excited about preparing these wonderful healthy dishes. Remember to keep your grocery shopping as basic as possible with emphasis on herbs and spices to create some truly unique flavors and avoid processed foods at all costs.

About the Author

Born in New Germantown, Pennsylvania, Stephanie Sharp received a Masters degree from Penn State in English Literature. Driven by her passion to create culinary masterpieces, she applied and was accepted to The International Culinary School of the Art Institute where she excelled in French cuisine. She has married her cooking skills with an aptitude for business by opening her own small cooking school where she teaches students of all ages.

Stephanie's talents extend to being an author as well and she has written over 400 e-books on the art of cooking and baking that include her most popular recipes.

Sharp has been fortunate enough to raise a family near her hometown in Pennsylvania where she, her husband and children live in a beautiful rustic house on an extensive piece of land. Her other passion is taking care of the furry members of her family which include 3 cats, 2 dogs and a potbelly pig named Wilbur.

Watch for more amazing books by Stephanie Sharp coming out in the next few months.

Author's Afterthoughts

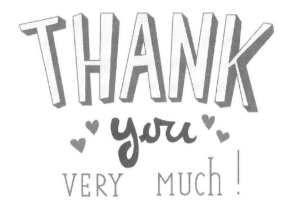

I am truly grateful to you for taking the time to read my book. I cherish all of my readers! Thanks ever so much to each of my cherished readers for investing the time to read this book!

With so many options available to you, your choice to buy my book is an honour, so my heartfelt thanks at reading it from beginning to end!

I value your feedback, so please take a moment to submit an honest and open review on Amazon so I can get valuable insight into my readers' opinions and others can benefit from your experience.

Thank you for taking the time to review!

Stephanie Sharp

For announcements about new releases, please follow my author page on Amazon.com!

(Look for the Follow Bottom under the photo)

You can find that at:

https://www.amazon.com/author/stephanie-sharp

or Scan **QR-code** *below.*

Made in the USA
Monee, IL
16 February 2020

616.9246 SHARP
Let us help you demystify Lyme Disease /
33772001165500
THORNTON   30May20